I Am Not a Bad Person

The Confession of a Cancer Cell

Please unleash your imagination while reading this book.

Because this book is not written about the real world, but it is also about the real world.

What do you think it is, it is what it is.

1

I'm a worker in the Initiator Factor workshop, specifically in Team F. There are other colleagues in my team. Our workplace consists of the Ribosome machine and the mRNA assembly line. The machine has three slots: A, P, and E, and two subunits of different sizes.

The initiation factor is a part of protein biosynthesis that provides influencing substances for cells. This is a anthropomorphic workshop.

Every day when the AUG light comes on, we start working.

Our job is to assemble tRNA parts carrying amino acids into the ribosome machine, then move the machine onto the pre-assembled mRNA on the front assembly line, and finally screw the parts onto the mRNA.

I've heard the assembled mRNA will be shipped to the next factory. They assemble into something huge, sustaining the world we live in. But I've never seen it because I've always been working in the factory.

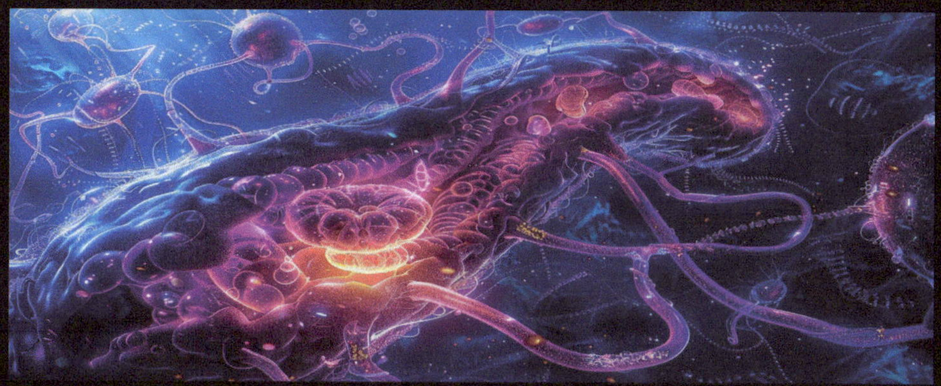

My job is the most technical but also the most tedious part. It's about matching each screw strictly according to the letters on them and the mRNA nuts. For example, the A screw can only match the U nut, and the C screw must align with G. My favorite screw is the I screw because it can match any nut except the G nut.

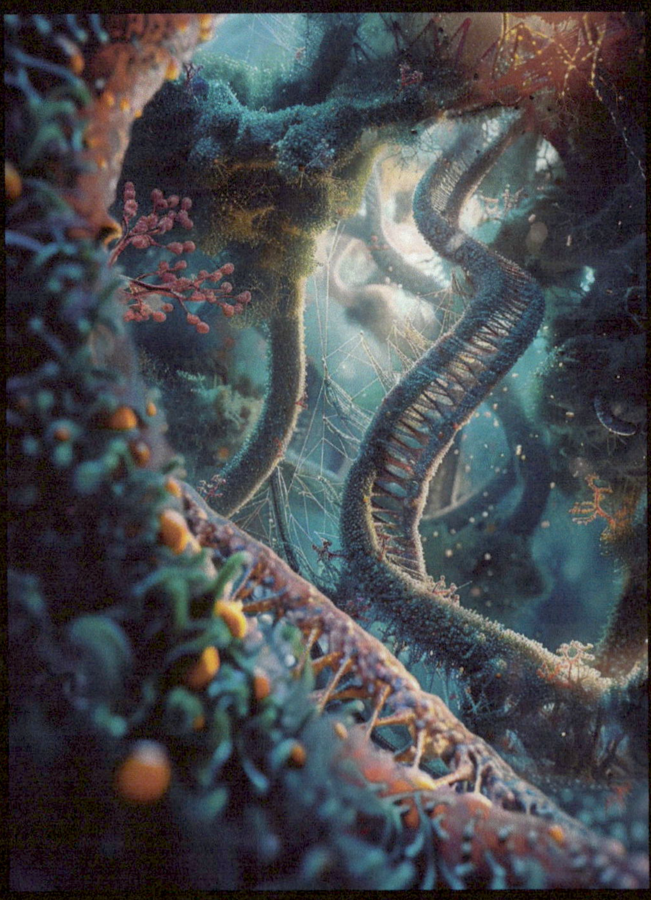

Of course, what I love most is seeing the UAG light come on because it means it's finally time to clock out.

I love my job. My ancestors have been working here for generations, so I'm here too.

Every day, we clock in and out, diligently screwing nuts and operating machines, and the days go by.

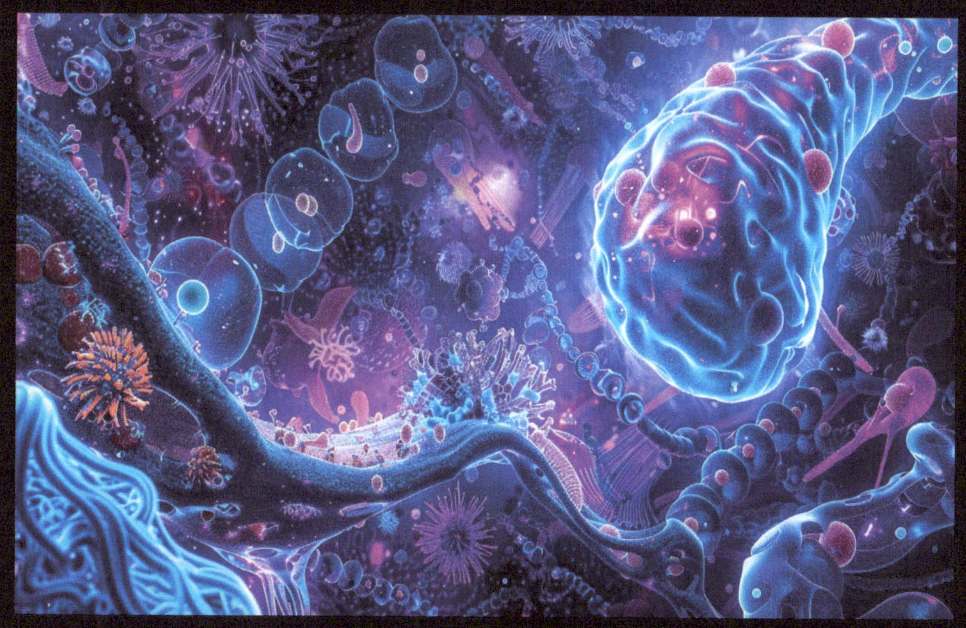

2

    Until one day, I discovered an error in my work, although I wasn't sure if it was my fault.

    I followed the nut pairing standards strictly, assembling each part diligently. However, the final assembly of the mRNA looked different from usual, with some parts appearing particularly strange.

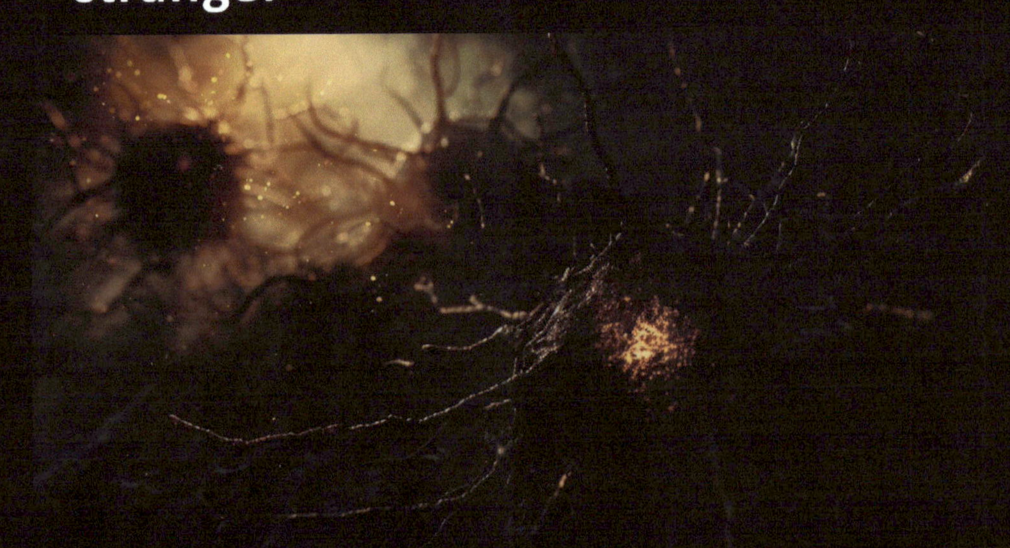

I quickly sought out **RB**, our quality supervisor, and explained the situation to him.

He promptly contacted other inspectors like **APC**, **P53**, and together, we convened a meeting.

We decided to report the issue to the headquarters DNA building and check if there were any errors in the nut sequences provided to us.

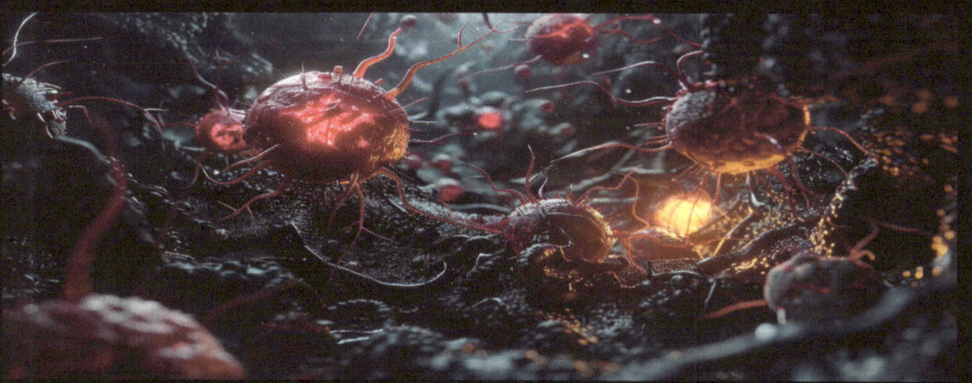

Such situations occurred frequently, but usually, after reporting to headquarters, most issues would be resolved.

However, this time seemed different.

When they returned, they informed me that there were no errors. They explained that this was a new product of production; the old-fashioned products were no longer meeting the demands. Therefore, headquarters made adjustments. It was a top-level mutation, but it wouldn't affect our factory.

We just needed to continue working according to the new requirements.

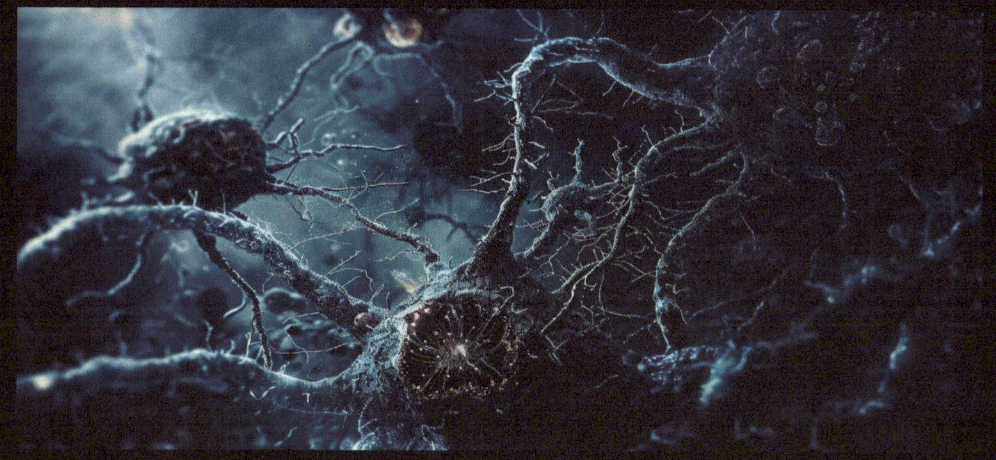

I worried that these changes might cause problems, but they suddenly rebuked me sternly.

I had no choice but to continue working diligently, trusting that if headquarters had confirmed there were no issues, then there shouldn't be any.

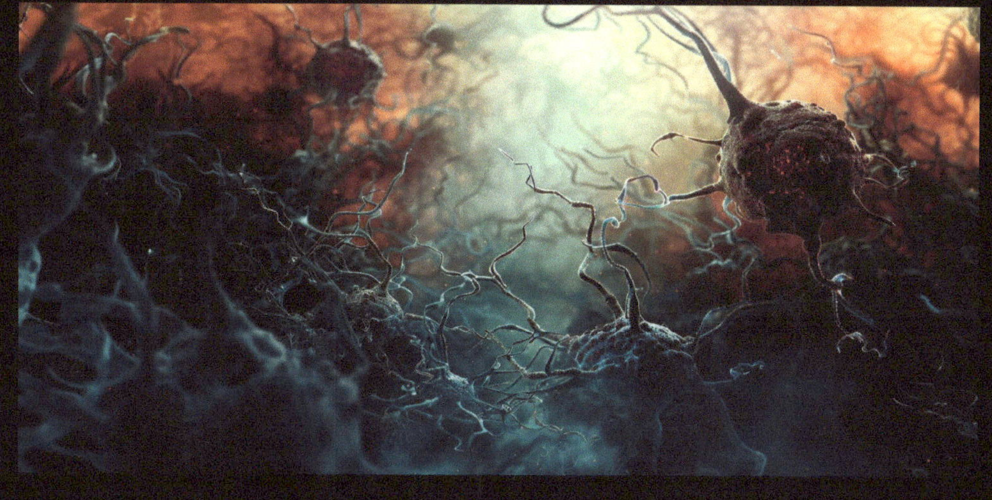

3

After some time passed, I noticed the situation was getting worse.

The mRNA we produced became increasingly strange, with more and more inconsistencies.

Then, headquarters sent over a guy named Ras. He was like a shot of adrenaline, working tirelessly day and night, pushing us to our limits.

We were exhausted every day, yet our pay kept decreasing, and our money couldn't buy much.

The ATP market often faced shortages, and life was getting worse day by day. But we had to keep working, assembling that bizarre machine.

It was getting stranger and uglier by the day.

One day, I found myself staring blankly at the banner overhead, which read, "*Work hard to create a better life.*" I muttered, questioning whether our work was truly creating a better life.

Suddenly, a voice behind me roared, "Are you questioning the correctness of headquarters?"

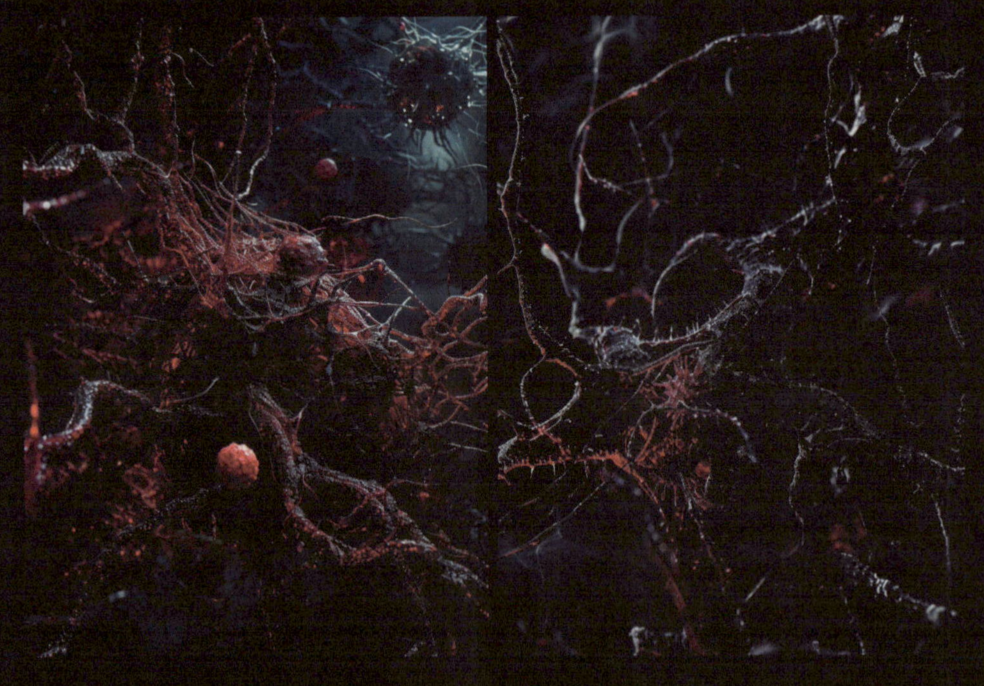

I turned around to see the **Macrophage** Guard, glaring at me with an lysosome gun in hand.

Fortunately, an old employee nearby intervened on my behalf, preventing further investigation.

In the end, the guard glared at me fiercely, warning that if I dared to express antigen skepticism again, he wouldn't hesitate to dissolve me on the spot.

Later, I heard they suspected there were infiltrators, but they couldn't catch them. So, they increased the number of guards, making the atmosphere extremely tense.

Macrophages are white blood cells located within tissues. Their main function is to phage cell debris and pathogens in the form of fixed or free cells.

4

Now I often feel afraid. What if these terrifying things, once shipped out, assemble into something that could harm us? Can it still help maintain our current living environment, or will it kill us all? Every time I think about this, I worry so much that I can't sleep.

Unfortunately, my fears have become reality.

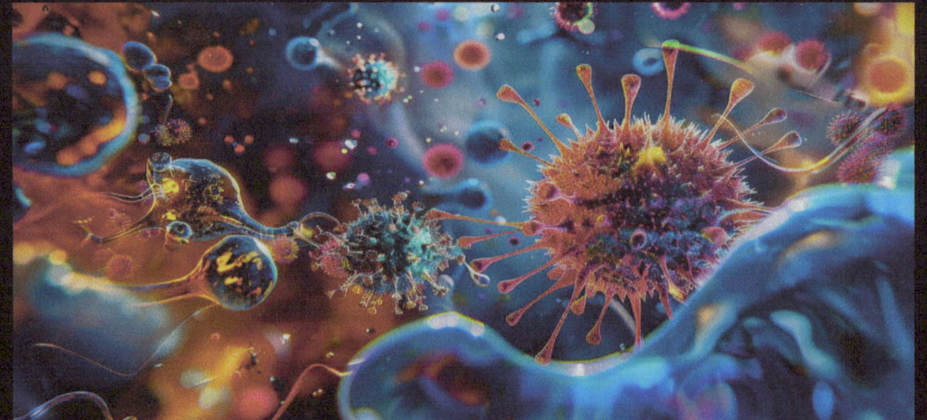

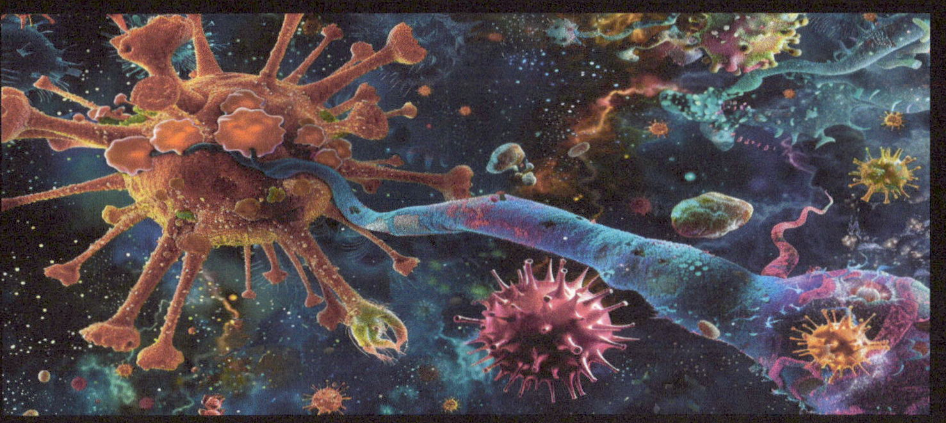

    Nowadays, we're forced to work every day without receiving any pay. The market has completely dried up, and we haven't eaten for days.

    The weather is getting colder, colder than it has ever been. I heard a few days ago that a vital energy pipeline nearby broke, but the reason remains unclear.

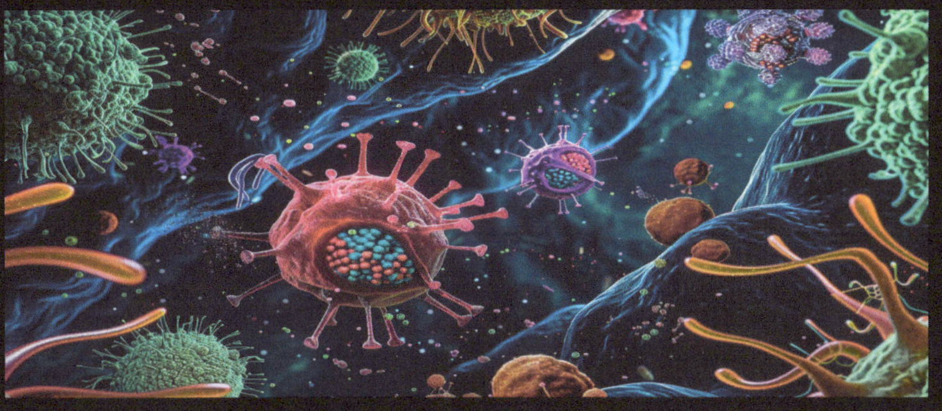

We have no choice but to approach the factory's leaders together to report the situation, hoping for an explanation and a resolution to the problem. But the replies we receive are always the same.

They say it's an order from DNA headquarters, telling us to continue working hard, assuring us that the difficulties will pass.

Pointing at the monstrous creature on the production line, we ask, "Is this normal? Look at it. Can something like this help us survive? It will only destroy us!"

An elder in the factory speaks up, "I've worked here my whole life, and I've never seen anything so terrifying. Why does headquarters want us to produce such things? Are they trying to destroy us all?"

Amidst the chaos, a mechanical voice echoes from the sky, "A pairs with U, C pairs with G, U pairs with AG, G pairs with UC, I pairs with ACU." It feels like a curse lingering in everyone's mind.

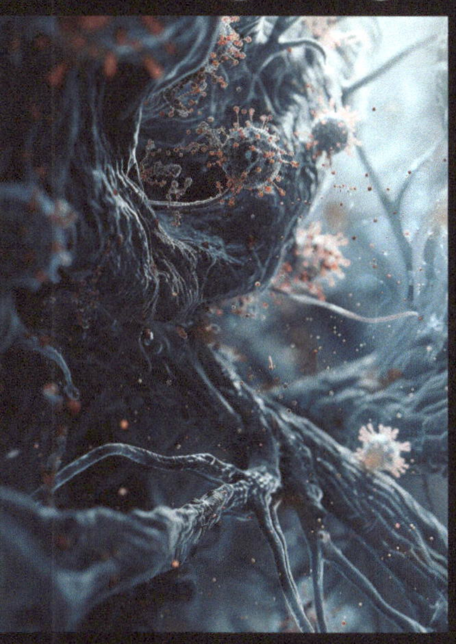
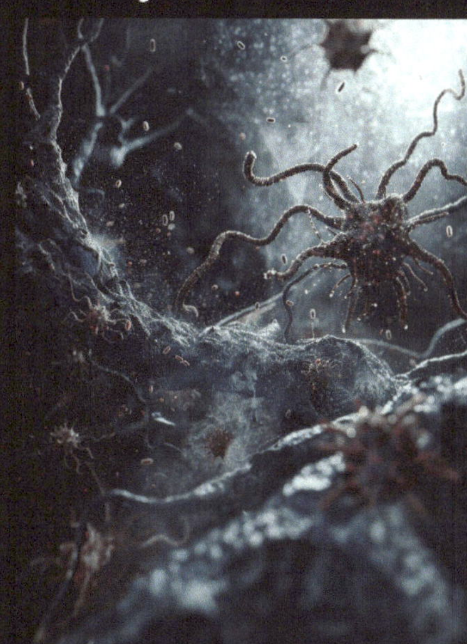

The voice repeats incessantly,
growing fainter and more distant,
as the sky darkens and the cold
intensifies.

Like everyone else, I return
helplessly to my workstation. I
don't know if I can endure this.

In my heart, I think, if things
continue like this, I might die...

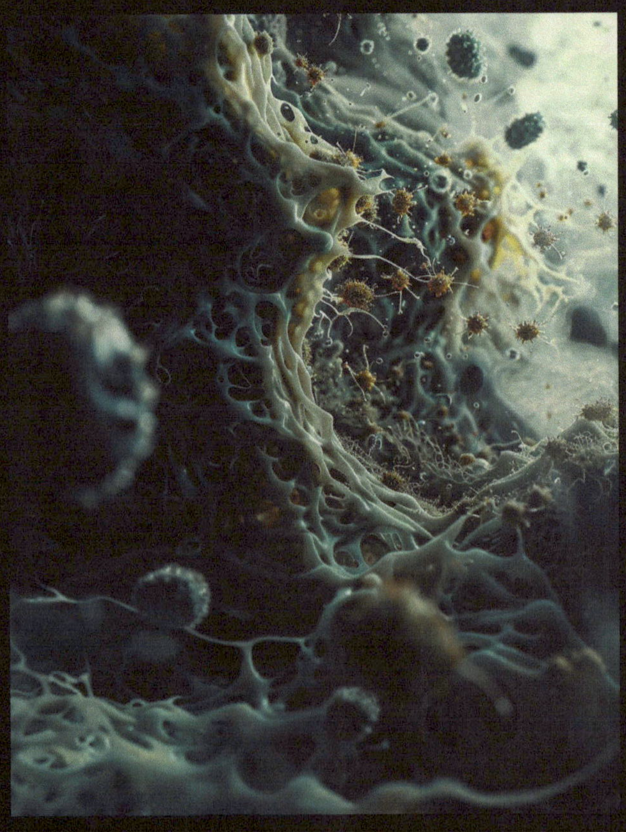

5

As time passed, we continued working on the production line every day. Our pay was sporadic, but thankfully, the ATP in the market was prioritized for us, ensuring we wouldn't starve and could continue assembling the monsters in front of us.

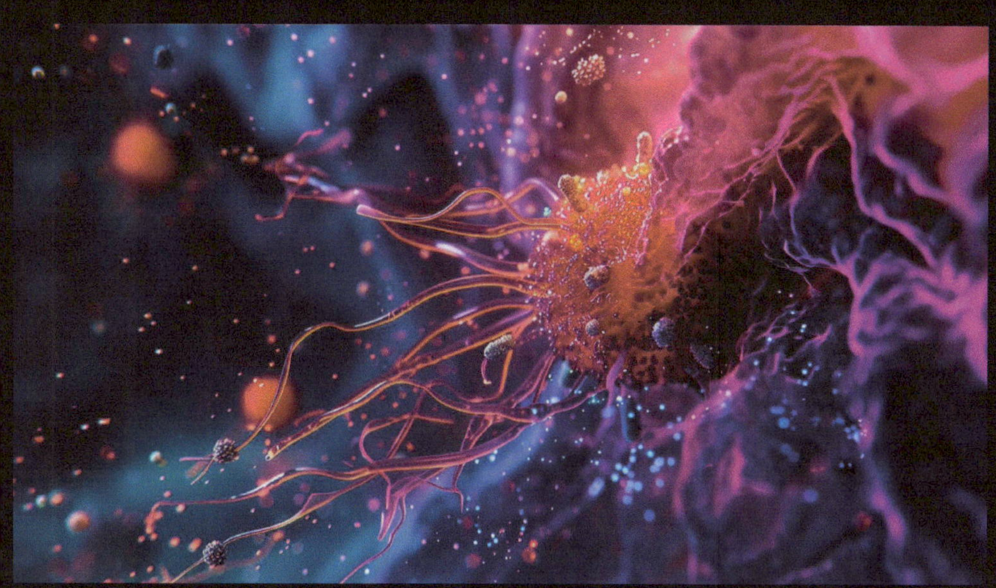

Leaders told us that infiltrators had entered our ranks, disguising themselves well. Despite daily patrols, the guards couldn't catch them. They continued causing damage, so we had to work even harder to repair the losses they caused.

Though we weren't sure if our efforts were effective, it was better than doing nothing at all.

Over time, we started privately discussing who could have such strong destructive abilities and why they would do this. Some even suspected they were fabricated to scare us into continuing to work.

Then one day, a group of strangers stormed into the factory like madmen, smashing our machines and injuring our workers.

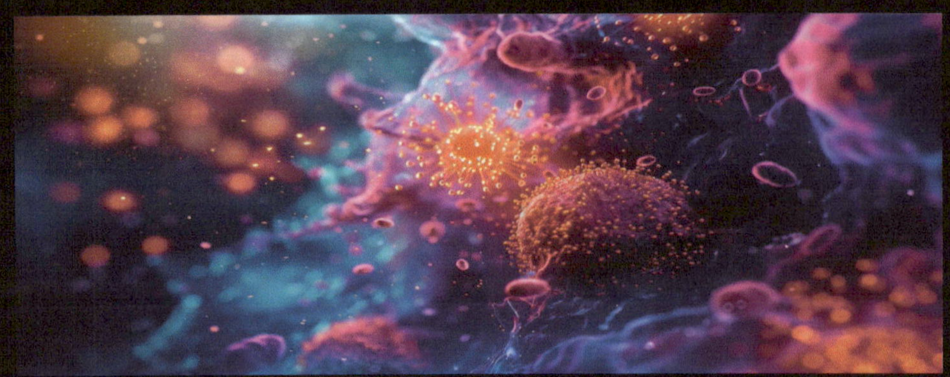

   We sought help from the guards, but **Captain T** said it wasn't their concern because these people didn't carry antigens and weren't the ones they were looking for. They had no authority to intervene, leaving us infuriated but powerless.

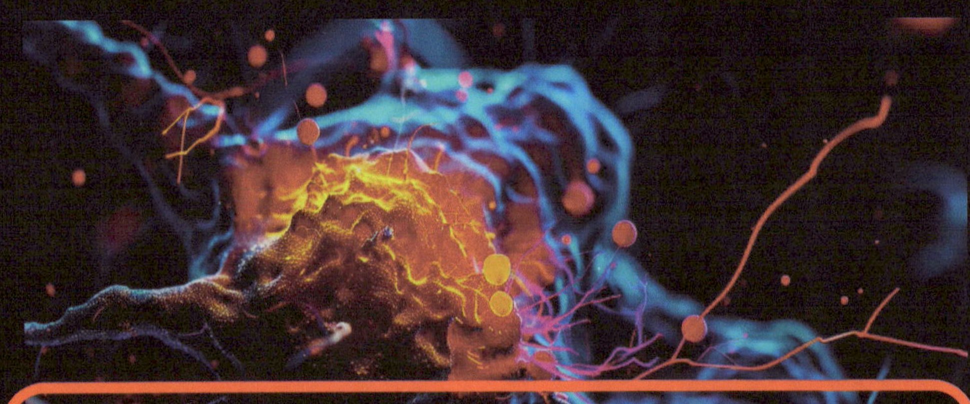

These individuals continued causing havoc behind the scenes, posing as our own, damaging our screws and nuts, disrupting our work. Especially a pair named 5-Fluorouracil and 6-Thioguanine, who looked so much like us, they often managed to infiltrate.

There was also one called Methotrexate, who liked stealing our tetrahydrofolate, depriving us of one-carbon fuel.

Their names were strange—things like Adenosine, Nitrosylserine—but they were exceptionally skilled at disrupting our production.

6

In such an environment, our factory was becoming increasingly unsustainable.

Then one day, the factory manager gathered us all and somberly informed us that the mob had breached and taken control of the headquarters building. They claimed to be the rightful authority, intending to overthrow the previous headquarters' orders, and they even gave us a new name: "Tumor."

They accused us of being the demons' henchmen, accomplices of death. They were the ones wreaking havoc in the factory and injuring our workers, yet they shifted the blame onto us, claiming we were the ones dragging the world down.

After a pause, the manager continued, his voice trembling slightly. He delivered the worst news: Since they now controlled headquarters, the guards were on their side, and they would soon come to arrest us.

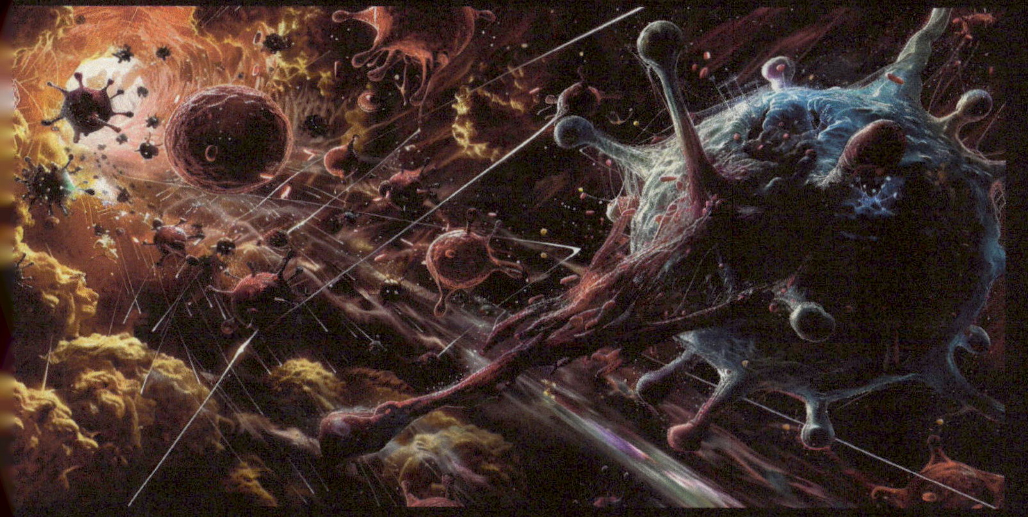

There was uproar among the crowd.

I was stunned. How could honest laborers like us suddenly become criminals?

Someone shouted, "Why should they arrest us? We don't know anything, we haven't done anything wrong. We were just following orders from above."

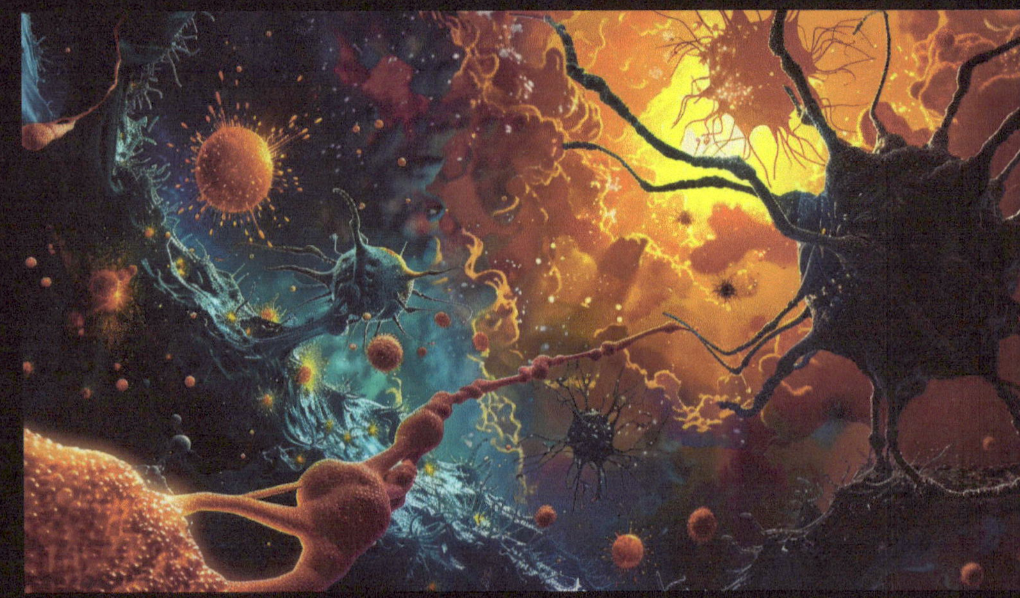

Yes, we were just ordinary workers, everything was arranged by that DNA bunch from headquarters. Why should they come after us? They should hold them accountable.

Every day, we toiled tirelessly to repair the damage, only to end up being labeled as villains. It was unfair!

Then someone suggested, "Manager, why don't we relocate? Go somewhere else and start afresh, build a new factory."

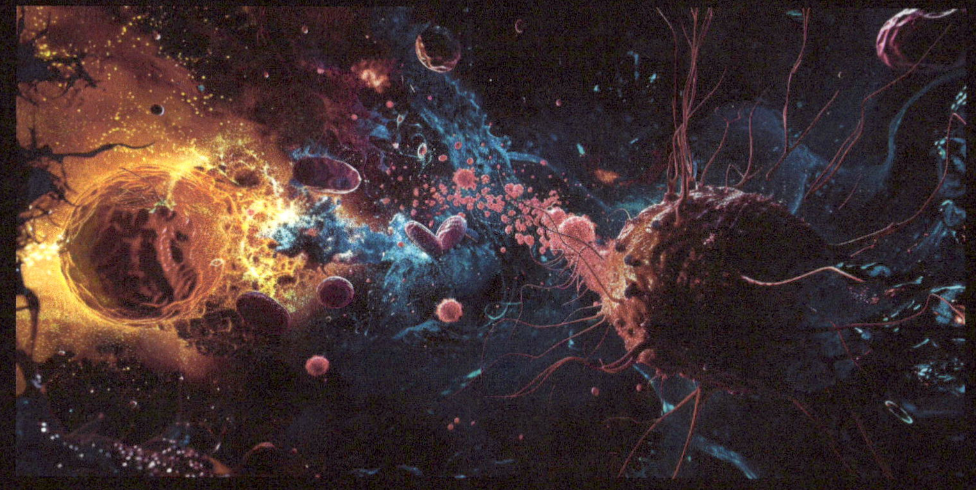

Many agreed.

The manager sighed heavily, taking a long time before responding, "Their people are everywhere. Where could we go? Without new mRNA provided by headquarters, what would we do? If we continue following the old standards, we'll surely be discovered and arrested sooner or later."

"And... and I've heard there's something called the basal membrane outside our factory, an obstacle we can never overcome."

With that, the manager's eyes scanned the crowd, and he said, "Unless..."

7

Just as the manager was about to continue speaking, there was suddenly a tremendous roar all around. The sky and the earth tore apart instantly, and the entire factory was ripped from the ground. If there were ever an apocalypse, I imagine it wouldn't be more terrifying than this.

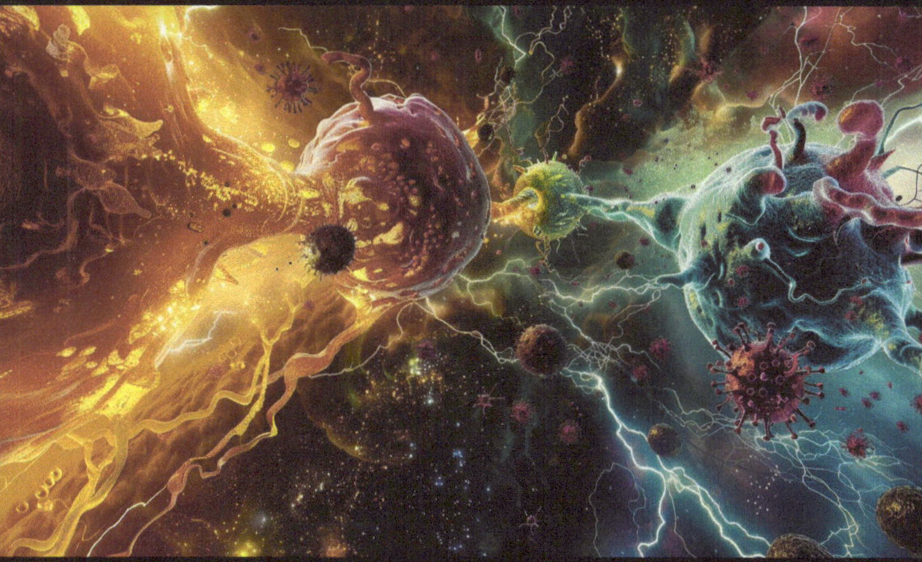

Almost everyone was seized by this external force. I struggled and ran out of the factory. Outside, the landscape was crumbling and collapsing, and the world before my eyes was falling apart.

Before I could think much, a massive object came crashing down, and I instantly lost consciousness.

I don't know how long it was before I faintly heard someone speaking nearby.

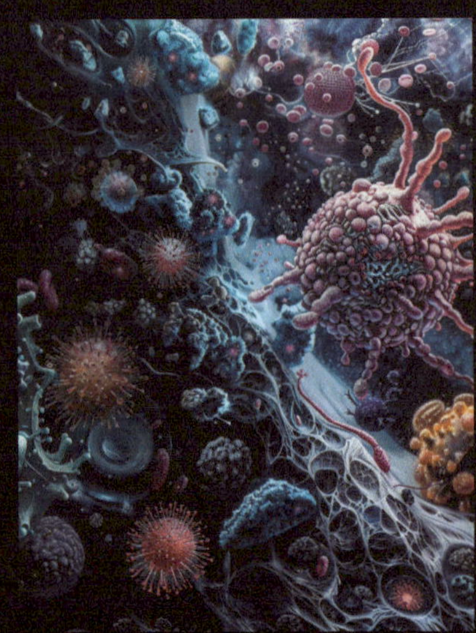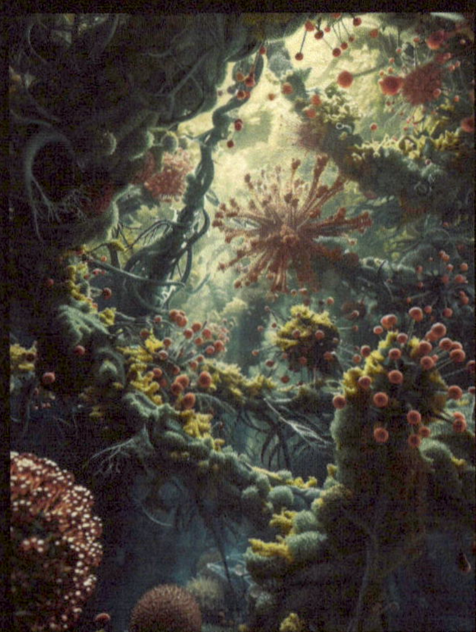

"He must have been the initiator factor from the original factory, but he seems a bit abnormal."

Another person said, "Anyway, he's still a protein. Let's ubiquitinate him."

Then I had a dream. I dreamt that I melted, turning into screws and small parts. Those tRNA molecules I used to manipulate every day carried my parts and flew onto the familiar assembly line.

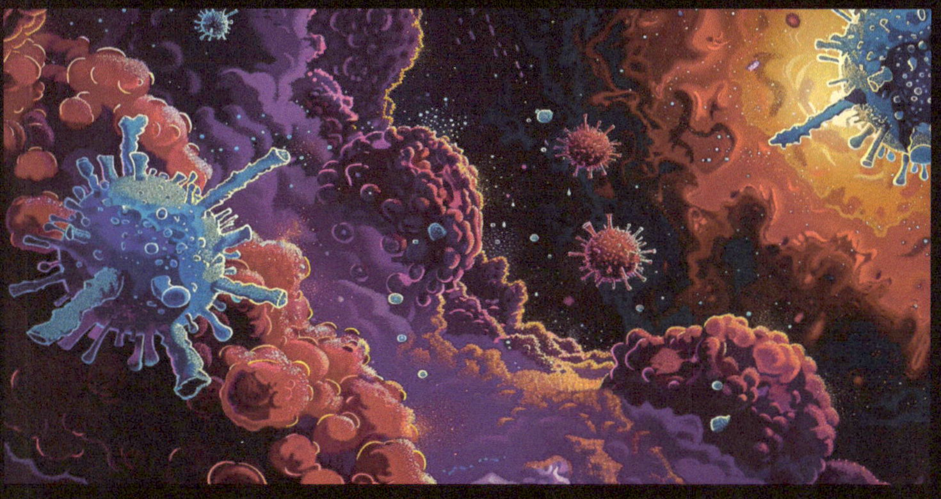

A guy like me, with a base-pairing table by his side, installed me bit by bit onto the mRNA.

Then, many assembled mRNAs gathered together, forming a colossal entity. I felt like I had finally arrived outside the factory.

Floating high in the air, I saw a completely different scenery

Our old factory site seemed to have turned into a giant crater. Everywhere, there were masses of flesh-like creatures, frantically busy repairing the damage.

Not far away, macrophage guards were running around arresting people. Strangely, they seemed to be getting bigger.

In the chaos, I spotted many factories identical to our previous one. They were scattered across the land, no, even in the sky.

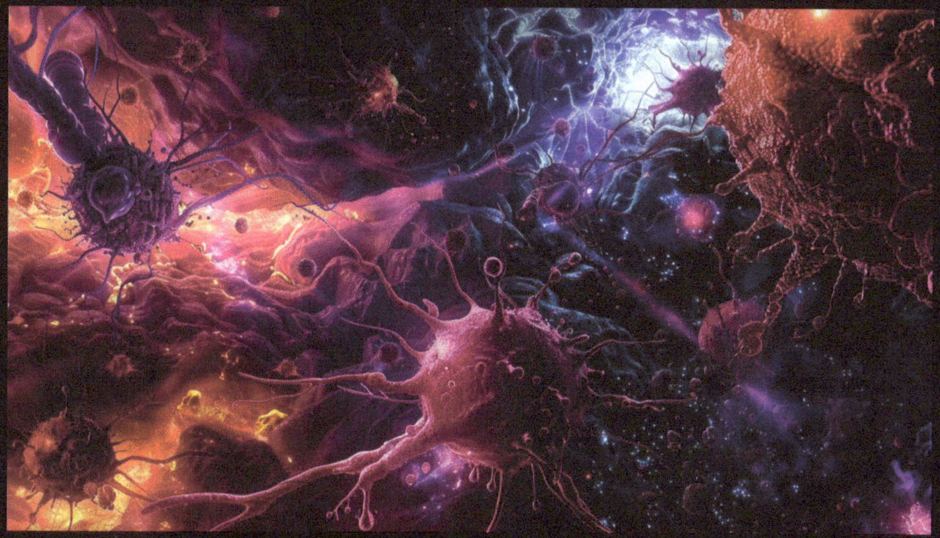

Countless little guys were tirelessly busy, just like we used to be. They linked together, stretching far into the distance until the boundary between heaven and earth blurred into one. Within them, the flashing AUG and UAG lights resembled the mesmerizing stars in the vast universe, pulsating with the rhythm of life.

At the farthest reaches of the flickering lights, I saw rows of towering structures, with double-helix-like patterns, as spectacular as I had heard, resembling the headquarters of DNA.

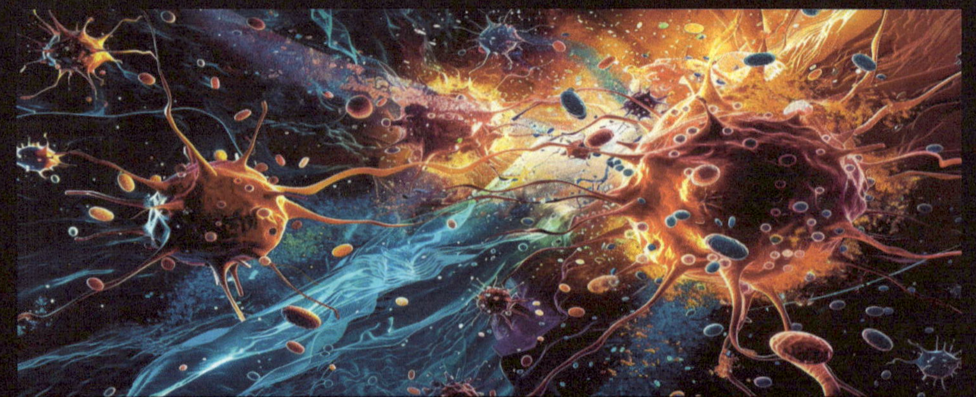

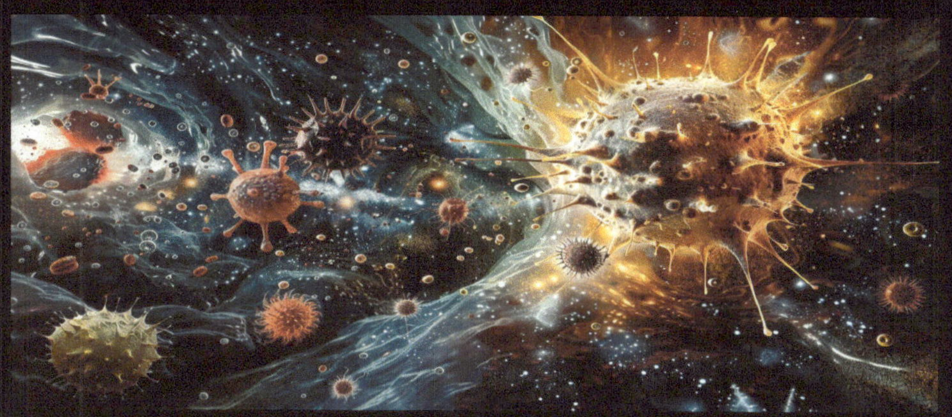

They unfolded and interwove, producing many familiar figures that flew into the flickering lights.

Looking at the scene before me, I didn't know if this was a dream or reality. Perhaps this was my afterlife. If it was a dream, I hoped I would never wake up.

I think... we made it through.

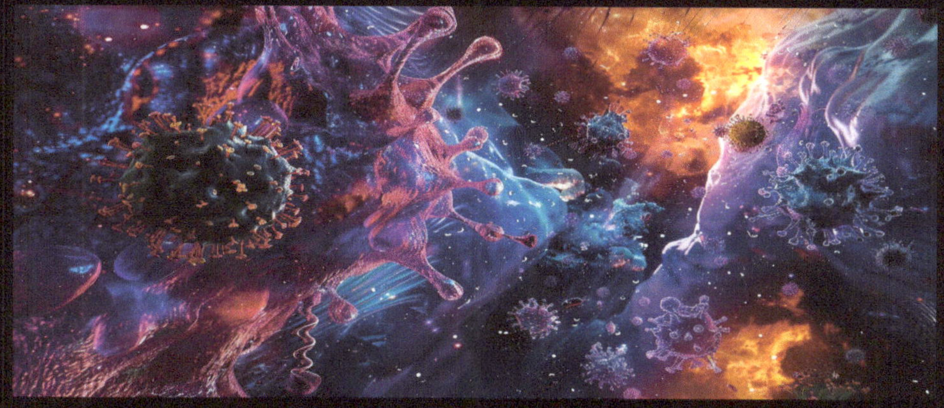

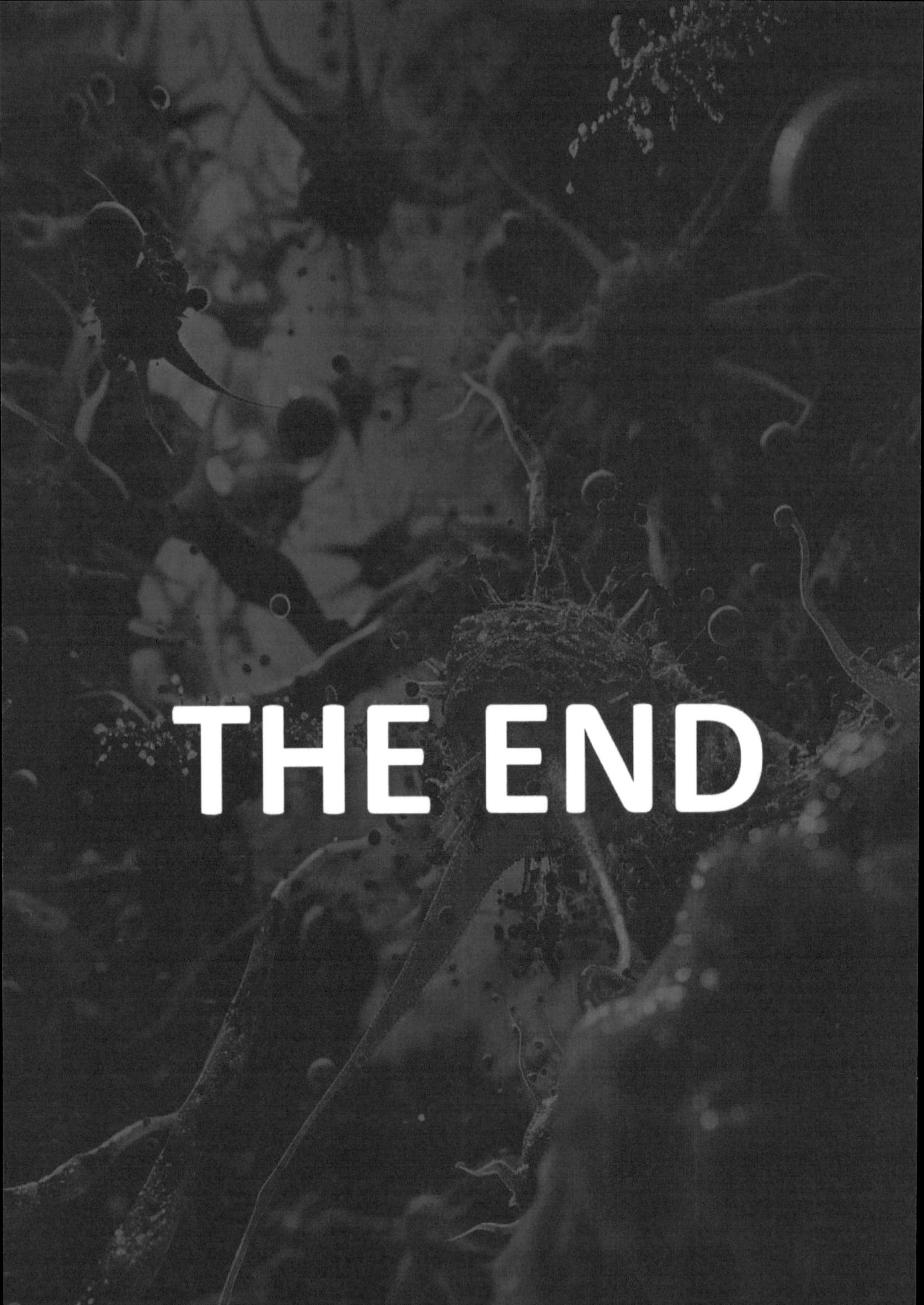

THE END

www.ingramcontent.com/pod-product-compliance
Lightning Source LLC
Chambersburg PA
CBHW040905260726
48664CB00025B/1507